# 50 TIPS
## TO BUILD YOUR
# CONFIDENCE

50 TIPS TO BUILD YOUR CONFIDENCE

Copyright © Summersdale Publishers Ltd, 2014

With research by Elanor Clarke

Summersdale Publishers Ltd
46 West Street
Chichester
West Sussex
PO19 1RP
UK

www.summersdale.com

Printed and bound in the Czech Republic

ISBN: 978-1-84953-508-3

Substantial discounts on bulk quantities of Summersdale books are available to corporations, professional associations and other organisations. For details contact Nicky Douglas by telephone: +44 (0) 1243 756902, fax: +44 (0) 1243 786300 or email: nicky@summersdale.com

# 50 TIPS
## TO BUILD YOUR
# CONFIDENCE

Anna Barnes

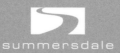

summersdale

# Introduction

When you think of a confident person, you may conjure up images of someone who is well presented, smiling, happy and comfortable talking in a crowd or addressing an audience. The fact is, though, the person in your mind's eye could still have inner confidence issues. Confidence is about believing in your abilities, and projecting this belief with your demeanour and actions, allowing others to see the best side of you. These easy-to-follow tips can help you understand what affects confidence, and learn how to build yours to a healthy level. If, however, you feel your confidence issues are strongly affecting your day-to-day life, it is recommended that you seek advice from your doctor.

# UNDERSTANDING CONFIDENCE

The key to being able to improve a situation is first to understand it. Knowing how low self-confidence can affect you, and being aware of your triggers, is a valuable way to start working on building your confidence.

# Keep a confidence diary

In order to understand your confidence issues, take some time to work out what your triggers are, and when your confidence is at its highest or lowest points. Choose a notebook that reflects your personality, be it a simple notepad or an illustrated diary, as you are more likely to want to pick up and use something you like the look of. Keep it where you are most likely to use it – by the bed, in the kitchen, wherever you think you will pick it up; but if you are concerned about a loved one delving into your notes, it could be kept in a drawer or cupboard that is easily accessible. The act of writing down how you feel, and what your confidence levels are like from day to day, will not only help you keep track of what may cause a bout of low confidence, it will also be cathartic. Remember to write down the high points as well as the lows; the diary will give you something to refer back to on low-confidence days, reminding you that things can be better.

# Know your triggers

Once you have been keeping your diary for a while, you are likely to start noticing some patterns. It may be that there are certain situations which always knock your confidence, or that talking to a certain friend always gives you a boost. The people and situations which cause your confidence levels to drop are known as 'triggers', and one of the simplest things you can do to help break this cycle of low confidence is to avoid them. A friend who makes you feel bad about yourself is not a true friend; a class which leaves you feeling low is not having a positive effect on your life. If you cannot completely avoid your triggers, then use the tips that follow as a means to cope with them and to gradually change them.

# See a more confident you

When starting out on a journey of self-improvement, it can be hard to see what the end result will be. It is easy to become bogged down in the 'what ifs' a situation brings to mind, and this is where visualisation can help. Sitting in a comfortable chair, in a relaxed position, close your eyes and begin to focus on your breathing. There is no need to breathe more slowly, just pay attention to your natural breathing patterns. Next, start to build a picture in your head of how a more confident you would look and act. Where are you? Who is with you? Notice the details and enjoy the feeling of confidence from within. While you are working on building your confidence, take this mental image with you and see it as something to look forward to.

## 4

# Where are you confident?

An important question to ask yourself is, where do you feel most and least confident? This is not just a question of location – although for some people certain places bolster their confidence or make them feel worse – it is more about the areas of your life you feel are at polar opposites where your confidence is concerned. Someone may, for example, feel that they have raised their family well, and be confident as a parent, whilst lacking in confidence when it comes to work. Knowing the areas, both physical and emotional, which affect your confidence can help you to build your confidence levels. At first, situations or places which knock your confidence can be avoided when it is already at a low point, and later you can work on altering the way you perceive and feel about these situations using the tips in this book, particularly those which emphasise mindfulness.

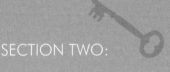

# SECTION TWO:

# EXERCISE FOR BODY CONFIDENCE

Feeling comfortable in your own skin is one of the most effective ways to boost your confidence. Regular exercise can help you achieve your goals both physically and emotionally. As well as toning your muscles, it helps relaxation and reduces stress, all adding up to a positive, confidence-building formula.

# Walk tall

Starting to exercise can be daunting, especially if your confidence is already rather low. Joining a gym or going to a group class can seem like the last thing you would want to do. However, exercise can be as simple as going for a walk. Just a half-hour walk each day can significantly improve your health and emotional well-being. You can fit this in on the way to work, at lunchtime or whenever feels right for you. The best walks are in daylight, in natural surroundings. Not only will being outdoors offer a natural boost, helping you feel better and lifting your spirits, but the exercise itself will also produce endorphins, making you feel great, and seeing your body shape start to improve is bound to give your confidence a lift.

# 6

# Swim towards a more confident you

Swimming is one of the most effective forms of exercise, both in terms of giving you a full-body workout and in allowing you to relax and unwind. The rhythmic lap of the water with each stroke, and the focus on your technique and breathing, really make this a great way to move your mind away from your worries, allowing some quality time to yourself. This alone time can give you a chance to reflect on the positive changes you are making. Add to that the fact that floating in water is a wonderfully soothing experience, and all part and parcel of a trip to the pool, and you've got a perfect recipe for confidence-boosting relaxation.

# 7

## Try t'ai chi

A 'moving meditation', t'ai chi is an ancient Chinese martial art but is non-combative. It is distinctive for its slow, precise movements, which help improve posture, balance, strength and flexibility. Furthermore, this ancient art is said to promote the healthy flow of energy, or 'qi', throughout the body and to calm the mind. The relaxation and focus that this softer martial art provides, as well as the fact that you do not have to worry about whatever level anyone else is at, can have a very positive effect on your confidence levels, as you feel refreshed, stronger and as though you are working towards your own personal goals.

# Get into gardening

As well as being a great way to burn calories, being in the garden is a form of 'green exercise' – activity which takes place in nature – which research shows has even more health and well-being benefits than, say, visits to the gym. Gardening can improve your mood, ease muscle tension and lower blood pressure. Feeling close to nature can give you the boost you need to keep calm under pressure, and the act of pruning, weeding, planting, and finally seeing something grow gives you something to look forward to and feel proud of, which is sure to raise your confidence levels.

# Yoga for inner and outer strength

The ancient practice of yoga is not just about bending your body, but also about bringing balance to your mind. Yoga is practised at your own pace, allowing you to take time to really understand what your body can do. It can help with confidence because of the strengthening and toning effect it has on the body, and because of the calming effect it has on the mind. Most classes will finish with yogic sleep, or guided meditation, which can leave you feeling refreshed, happier and more in touch with yourself. If you would rather not attend a class, yoga can be practised at home with the help of books, DVDs or online demonstrations.

SECTION THREE:

# FUEL YOUR CONFIDENCE

Feeding your body the right balance of foods, and ensuring you include mood-boosting nutrients, is a great way to fuel your confidence from the inside out.

## 10

# Eat a balanced diet

Before we look at the specific nutrients that can be beneficial to confidence, it is important to ensure you have a balanced diet. Eating the right amount of calories for your age, height and sex, and ensuring you get enough proteins, fibre and vitamin-rich fruit and vegetables, whilst avoiding too many refined foods, will give you a good basis for general health and well-being. It should also improve digestion, which will make you feel healthier overall.

# Say no to alcohol

When feeling low, for example after a hard day at work, or when lacking confidence in a social situation, many people will reach for a drink to help them relax. Alcohol does have an instantly calming effect, but this is negated by the depressant qualities of alcohol, and the feeling of anxiety that can be left behind once the effects wear off. Alcohol can also disturb your sleep, contrary to the popular idea of a 'nightcap'. Try to cut down your drinking as much as possible, and if you do go for a tipple, opt for a small glass of Chianti, Merlot or Cabernet Sauvignon, as the plant chemicals called procyanidins, which are abundant in these particular wines, are beneficial to health, especially cardiovascular health. These wines are also rich in melatonin, the sleep hormone, and a well-rested person is more likely to be a confident person.

## 12

# Learn to love whole grains

Whilst it can be easy to reach for a cake or biscuit in times of need, the refined flour and sugar combination in these foods can be detrimental to health and cause a wide variety of problems, from poor skin condition to serious illnesses such as diabetes, all of which are bound to have a negative effect on your confidence levels. Instead, try to include more whole grains in your diet. This can be as simple as switching white bread for wholemeal, white rice for whole rice, or choosing a breakfast cereal which contains whole grains. You could also try some of the many interesting grains available by getting creative with your cooking – why not try using quinoa in a salad, or bulgur wheat with a tagine – the combinations are endless.

# Perk up with proteins

Lean proteins such as chicken, fish or tofu are a key part of a healthy diet and work as confidence boosters in several ways. Firstly, they keep you feeling fuller for longer, therefore allowing you to eat more sensibly and feel a sense of achievement at improving your diet. Secondly, their amino acids help form neurotransmitters such as serotonin, dopamine and noradrenaline, which balance mood and keep you feeling positive. Finally, a protein-rich diet allows for quality healing and muscle building after exercise, helping you to move towards the body you want and body confidence.

14

# Learn about good fats

When trying to eat healthily, it can be easy to see fat as the enemy. Many 'healthy' products are marketed as low fat or fat-free, and we are led to believe that fat makes you fat. This is not entirely true. Fats are an important part of your diet. They are key in neurotransmitter production due to the amino acids they contain, and unsaturated fats are important for healthy skin and hair, which in turn will make you feel more confident about yourself. As long as you get the balance right, and are eating plenty of monounsaturated and polyunsaturated fats such as those found in olive oil and seeds, and you are reducing the amount of saturated fat you consume, for example the fats in butter, cheese and red meat, you will start to feel the benefits.

# Cut down on caffeine

Caffeine and other similar stimulants should be avoided as much as possible. Many of us rely on that first cup of coffee in the morning to wake us up, or a cup of tea to keep us going at midday, but these caffeinated drinks – along with cola and foods containing caffeine, such as chocolate – could be having an adverse effect on your confidence by increasing your stress levels.

Having a caffeinated drink can make us feel more alert because it induces the initial stages of the stress reaction, boosting cortisol production. Consuming large quantities of caffeine, however, can cause the exhaustion phase of stress and lead to anxiety, which can have a very negative impact on confidence levels. Added to this, caffeine can be very addictive and stopping suddenly can cause withdrawal symptoms, which can make you feel physically unwell and emotionally under pressure – not a good combination for confidence. Try cutting down slowly to no more than 300 mg of caffeine a day, that's the equivalent of three mugs of coffee or four mugs of tea. Have fun experimenting with the huge variety of herbal teas and decaffeinated coffees and teas available on the market, and notice the improvement in your mood and ability to cope.

# Be ACE

Low confidence can make the body feel stressed, and high levels of stress hormones in your system can have a negative effect on your health, either by lowering your immune system, making you more prone to coughs, colds and other infections, or by over-stimulating it and provoking autoimmune illnesses and inflammation. A simple way to combat these symptoms is to eat plenty of foods rich in the antioxidant vitamins A, C and E. These antioxidants help normalise the body and reduce inflammation, whilst boosting immunity.

Vitamin A is found in the form of retinol in products such as fish liver oil and egg yolks.

Too much retinol can be bad for health though, so balance this with beta-carotene, found in mainly yellow and orange fruits and vegetables such as carrots, butternut squash and apricots. Vitamin C is found in good amounts in citrus fruits, broccoli, berries and tomatoes, and vitamin E is found in nuts, seeds, avocados, olive oil and wheatgerm. Adding some of these foods to your diet could make you feel healthier and happier, as well as improving the look of your skin and hair, which can help with body confidence.

# LESS STRESS =
# MORE CONFIDENCE

Do you ever feel you just can't keep up? Like your abilities just aren't enough to help you stay on top of everything? We lead ever-busier lives and this can in turn cause ever-rising stress levels. Feeling stressed can lead to confidence issues, particularly if you feel like you are not doing well enough considering how tired or overworked you feel. Try these stress-busting tips to help pull your stress levels down and your confidence levels up.

# Write away your worries

Everyone will have periods of worry at some point – family, finance, career and health can all be sources of anxiety. Not being able to 'switch off' and continuing to worry about several different things at once can make us feel out of control and therefore knock our confidence. Writing these worries down allows you to voice them, helping you to think more clearly and allowing you to relax more easily. Some people find a further step helpful: if you destroy the paper the worries are listed on by, for example, either ripping it up or throwing it into a fire, you can actually see your worries move from your head, to the paper and then away.

# Practise mindfulness

Mindfulness, which has developed from Buddhist teachings, is a technique for living in the here and now, rather than being preoccupied with the past or the future. Stop worrying about what you have or haven't done and all the things you still have to do. Being mindful means living in the moment and truly experiencing what is happening now. A simple way to start would be by altering your route to work slightly so that you pay more attention to your surroundings, rather than being on autopilot.

Taking time to reflect on your environment and situations can put your worries into perspective, where otherwise they might have preoccupied you and caused you stress. Furthermore, you will be paying more attention to the positive aspects of your day and will be more likely to see the areas in which you are doing well. Just seeing that these areas exist can be a huge confidence boost.

## 19

# Keep it simple

Having too many things going on around you at once can be a major cause of stress, and can give your confidence a knock, particularly if you feel like you cannot get through all the tasks ahead of you. One key example of this is clutter; having too much 'stuff' around you can cause stress as there is always something to think about, something to put away, something to clean (cleaning is harder, too, with so many items to move and clean under or around). Furthermore, this excess of things can make it hard to concentrate on the task at hand, as it causes distractions. De-cluttering, throwing out old items that are no longer of use and giving them to a charity shop or using sites such as Freecycle and eBay is a great first step to simplifying your life, leaving you feeling more in control, less stressed, and more confident in your ability to look after yourself and your home.

# Talk to a friend or family member

If you think stresses and worries are affecting your confidence, talking to someone close to you can be a huge help. Vocalising your concerns, and hearing the reassurance and advice of someone whose opinions you trust, can alleviate anxiety and let us see that we are not alone. If you do not have someone to confide in, a counsellor or a service such as the Samaritans can provide the sympathetic ear you seek. The simple act of picking up the phone to talk to someone takes faith and demonstrates that you can be a confident, open person.

# Avoid 'catching' stress from your colleagues

For many, the workplace is the most stressful area of their lives. A large amount of workplace stress is so-called 'second-hand' stress. When a colleague is feeling stressed you can unconsciously absorb their feelings of negativity. To avoid this, if a colleague is talking about work or personal problems, try to say something positive about the subject or offer them some advice. If they carry on, perhaps go to make a hot drink, or, if you cannot walk away, make sure you stay positive and try your best not to adopt your colleague's mindset. It takes faith to challenge a colleague's negativity, so as well as reducing stress, this can boost your confidence by showing you that you are capable of taking up such a challenge.

## 22

# Keep spending sensible

Financial worries are one of today's biggest stressors, with more and more people in debt and/or out of work. Taking control of your finances is a great confidence boost as it helps reduce the stress that can bring your confidence levels down, and it shows that you can take a situation on and improve it. Thankfully, there are some simple ways to cut back on non-essential spending.

Cancel any direct debits for services you do not want or need, for example, do you have a film club membership or subscriptions you hardly use? Next, look at debt – make sure you are paying off the debts with the highest interest rates first, so as to save money on interest. If you have a lot of credit card debt, now might be the time to take drastic action and cut up your maxed-out credit card – that way you can pay it off and not run up more debt.

Finally, it is important that when you do spend your money, it is on the things that are important to you and make you happiest. For example, is your weekly night out with friends high on your list? If so, make sure you put some money aside for it. Is your car important to you? If not, you could cut the cost of running it by using public transport to get around.

# MAKE PLANS AND ACHIEVE YOUR GOALS

Keeping on top of what there is to do at home, at work and in our social lives can be overwhelming. Planning and staying organised allows you to take control, and therefore feel more confident in your day-to-day life.

# Try a to-do list

Simple as it may sound, if you are unsure about your organisational skills, then a to-do list may well be the best thing to try. It can seem like there is too much to do and not enough hours in the day. This may be true, but getting organised will help you feel confident in your ability to prioritise tasks and get them done on time. A simple notepad will suffice, or you could even invest in an attractive notebook to write your lists in, as if you take pleasure in this simple task it will encourage you to continue the habit. The to-do lists can be as simple or as detailed as you like; the main thing is that they work well for you, and that you enjoy ticking off each task as you complete it as an indication of achievement.

**24**

# Be prepared for the day ahead

The pressure of deadlines, meetings, phone calls and working long hours can all build up and cause us to doubt our ability to handle things, which can upset confidence levels. This can not only get in the way of an enjoyable, effective working life, but can also have a negative impact on the rest of your life.

A simple way to reduce this feeling of pressure is to plan and prepare for your working day. Pack your lunch the night before so that you are not rushing to put it together in the morning. Look up bus or train times in advance to ensure you know about any delays, and make a list of the tasks you wish to complete the day before, so when you get to your place of work, your day is already planned out. Taking these steps can give you more confidence in your workload management.

# Set goals which suit you

Goal setting is key to success, and therefore to confidence building. It may be that you want to set small goals to help break down bigger tasks into more comfortable chunks, or it may be that you have long-term aims that you want to make reality. The most important thing, no matter how big or small the goal, is that it suits your needs, lifestyle and interests. Your goal can be related to any aspect of your life. Do you want to learn to paint? Travel somewhere exotic? Learn a language? Now is the time to start. If you choose to do something because you feel you 'should', or because it is the socially acceptable goal for someone in your current position, the chances are you will not have the motivation to make it all the way. Instead, make sure your aims reflect what you really want and see how easily you work towards these goals that focus on your own happiness.

## 26

# Ensure your goals are SMART

Now that you have identified the goals which you feel will make you happy, why not try a further step to boost how effectively you work towards them? One positive way to ensure that your goals will work for you is by making them SMART (specific, measurable, attainable, relevant and time-bound). This can be applied to goals relating to any aspect of your life, and doesn't have to be work related. It means that you should know exactly what it is you want to achieve (S), you should be able to measure your progress (M), it should be possible for you to achieve it, though not too easy (A), it should relate to your wider goals (R) and you should know when you want to have reached your goal by (T). Why not try setting yourself some SMART goals in the notes pages at the end of this book?

# Strive towards your goals

You may be thinking, with all the planning in the world, there is no way all your goals are achievable. Or that your SMART goals just aren't smart enough. It is natural to have concerns, especially if your confidence is particularly low, but all obstacles can be overcome with discipline and determination. Think about how good you will feel when you reach your goal and use that as fuel when obstacles spring up. For example, if you are trying to achieve a better body shape, but you always have coffee and cake with a friend on Wednesdays, then try switching the cake to a fruit salad. If you feel your friend will be unsupportive, try spending time with a different friend. There are always ways to work around problems, and the feeling you get solving them, as well as moving steadily towards your goals, is bound to improve your confidence levels.

# TREAT YOURSELF WELL, FEEL WELL

With the busy lives we lead, it can be easy to stop being as kind to ourselves as we should be. Treating yourself well helps you look great on the outside as well as relaxing and refreshing you, making you feel good on the inside.

28

# Treat your hair

Having well-looked-after hair, just like having glowing skin, is an excellent way to boost your body confidence. Make sure you wash and condition regularly with products designed for your hair type: dry, oily, coloured or curly. If you feel in need of a bigger boost, why not invest in a hair masque to pamper yourself with, or try out a new haircut to represent the new direction you are taking. Be daring and show your personal style, and feel your confidence building.

## 29

# Get the glow

Glowing, healthy skin is the basis for feeling good about the way you look. Looking in the mirror and seeing a healthy complexion can have a very positive effect on confidence levels. Put simply, when you look good, it is more likely you will feel good. To keep your skin in the best shape, make sure you cleanse and moisturise regularly. You don't need to buy expensive products as cheaper brands contain the same ingredients. Just ensure that the product is designed for your skin type, e.g. dry, oily, combination or normal.

Another important factor to remember is sunscreen. Whilst it is easy to remember to bring out the suncream on a hot day, the truth is that it should be worn most of the time. The easiest way to protect your skin is to use a daytime moisturiser with added SPF. Getting a little time in the sun, however, is good for you. Up to 15 minutes without suncream will not only feel great on your skin, but will also help to boost your vitamin D levels, which in turn improves mood.

# Dress to impress

Does your current wardrobe leave something to be desired? If you have de-cluttered, now might be the time to replenish with clothes which flatter and make you feel good. The way you dress affects the way you feel, from the colours you choose to how an item fits. The old adage says 'dress for the job you want, not the one you have'. Choose clothes that fit well and reflect your personality. Make sure that when you look in the mirror, what you are wearing makes you think 'yes, I look good today', rather than 'what am I wearing' or 'it will have to do'. Feeling good in your clothes will make you feel more comfortable in yourself, and boost your confidence levels both in the workplace and socially.

# Make bath time sacred

A soak in the bath does wonders. As well as keeping you clean and fresh, a warm bath with your favourite bubbles or oils helps relax tense muscles and prepares the body for sleep – and being well-rested boosts confidence levels. Make the most of your bath; invest in some bath products which make you feel good, light some candles and maybe take a book with you to read whilst you soak. Take the time to let yourself really relax into the water and use your favourite body wash to cleanse away the day. This treat will make you feel more in tune, and help you feel better both physically and emotionally.

If you don't have a bathtub, or if it's a particularly hot day, a long, luxurious shower can give you the same benefits. The water on your skin can invigorate and refresh, and washing with your favourite shower gel or scrub, enjoying the scent of it on your skin, can give your confidence a real boost.

# SLEEP BETTER, FEEL BETTER

It can be hard to find motivation when sleep-deprived, and many aspects of our lives can fall by the wayside, leading to lack of confidence in our abilities. Being well-rested makes us feel calmer, more confident and improves concentration, so why not give your bed time routine a shake-up and see what good comes of it?

# Make your bedroom your sanctuary

Experts say that our bed should be for sleeping and sex only. Keeping the bed as a work- and life-stress-free zone will help your body and mind to identify it as a place of rest, relaxation, enjoyment and, ultimately, sleep. To achieve this, it is a good idea to free your room of computers and televisions – anything that will make you tempted to watch some late-night videos – and make your bedroom tidy and inviting; a safe, cocoon-like environment. Do paperwork in another room, and keep important discussions out of the bedroom. You'll soon be sleeping more soundly and reaping the benefits.

## 33

# Know how much sleep you need

When it comes to bedtime, understanding how much sleep is normal for you is the first step to better-quality sleep. Many of us lie awake at night worrying that we won't get the recommended eight hours' sleep that we need to function well. However, studies have shown that most people will have no problem functioning with six or seven hours' sleep, and furthermore, many find that if you have lost sleep, you only need to catch up about a third of the lost time to feel better; so, for example, if you went to bed an hour and a half late one night of the week, a 30-minute lie-in at the weekend should do the trick.

Changing our perceptions of the time we need to sleep can help us feel more secure, and therefore help us sleep more easily, with a better quality of sleep, which leaves us more rested and ready to take on new challenges with a positive outlook.

# Choose bed linen that makes you feel good

Just like your newly updated wardrobe, having bed linen which suits you and makes you feel good is a great confidence booster. As well as the benefit to your quality of sleep, attractive linen helps make your bedroom a place you can feel comfortable in. There is more to it than that, though.

Choosing the right bed linen for you means choosing something that will make you feel ready to sleep in the evening, and fresh and ready to go in the morning. For some people, cool cotton sheets and duvet covers work best. Others find silk gentler against their skin. For many people, synthetics make them sweat too much in the night, which can cause night-time waking, leaving you unrefreshed and even jittery. Invest in a couple of sets of good linen, rather than multiple cheap and cheerful sets of polyester sheets, and see how much difference it makes to how you feel about your bedroom.

# Keep your room cool and dark

Although many describe sleep as warm and comfortable, being too warm will make it difficult for you to stay asleep and will leave you feeling unrefreshed. Avoid leaving the heating on in your bedroom, even on very chilly evenings, as this will make the air too warm and you may become sweaty in the night. If possible, leave a window slightly open to allow the cool night air to moderate your room temperature. If this proves too noisy, perhaps a quiet fan or more lightweight bedding will do the trick. Your bedroom should only be around 16°C, and well ventilated, helping you sleep restfully through the night and wake feeling ready for the day ahead.

Light is another cause of disturbed sleep and early waking. While darkness causes your brain to produce melatonin, a hormone that makes you feel sleepy, light helps it produce serotonin, too much of which will make you feel more awake. To help keep your bedroom as dark as possible, make sure any electrical items such as stereos are turned off, not on standby, as the lights from their displays may keep you awake. Preferably you will have already removed them from your bedroom. You could also choose thick, dark curtains or blackout blinds to ensure outside light does not intrude and wake you.

# Progressive relaxation

Just like meditation and yoga, progressive relaxation is an excellent sleep aid. It is often the case that when low mood strikes and our confidence has dipped, we lie awake at night unable to relax. This exercise removes the pressure, breaking relaxation down into smaller steps. Start at your feet and work your way up your body, concentrating on one body part at a time. For each body part, clench it as tightly as you can before letting it go and feel the physical relaxation that comes with this release. Some people find it helpful to use a verbal aid, for example by saying or thinking 'I am relaxing my feet, my feet are now completely relaxed' and repeating for each body part.

SECTION EIGHT:

# THE POWER OF YOUR MIND

Your thoughts have a strong influence on the way you feel and behave. The tips in this section show ways to challenge your thoughts, and build a more positive self-image to help boost your confidence and self-belief.

# Recognise that a thought is just a thought

We each have as many as 50,000 thoughts every day. These can be banal like 'I wonder what's for dinner', or they can be powerful, such as 'I'm not good enough'. Part of the concept of mindfulness is recognising thoughts and seeing that they do not need to control the way you feel and behave. Repeating the same negative thought pattern for many years may have had a detrimental effect on your confidence levels, but once you can recognise this negativity as simply a thought, with no substance, you can begin to challenge it and rebuild your self-concept.

# Ask yourself 'why?'

One of the key ways to challenge negative thoughts that drain your confidence is to ask 'why?'. For example, the commonly held negative thought 'I'm not good enough' can make you worried about many aspects of your life; perhaps you feel you are not good enough at your job, not a good enough friend, not a good enough homemaker. Now is the time to ask yourself why that is: can you find five empirical reasons why you are not good enough? It is unlikely you can. Let logic prevail, if the only way you can answer this simple question is with 'because I know it's true' or with minor incidents from the past, you can begin to change your self-perception.

# Would you say it to a friend?

Coming to terms with the above exercise can be particularly hard if your confidence is at an all-time low, because you may strongly believe the thought you are trying to challenge. You may even find reasons, however spurious, that it is 'true'. In this case, try this: think about your best friend, sibling or colleague; somebody you respect. Now, would you tell this other person what you are telling yourself? The likelihood is that your answer is no. You may even be shocked at the thought; why would you treat someone that way? The answer is, you already do: yourself. The lesson here is to treat yourself like your best friend. Allow yourself the same consideration you would another person and be kind to yourself.

# Use mantras

A mantra is a positive phrase which you repeat to yourself, confirming your positive thoughts with affirmations, such as 'I am' or 'I will' instead of 'I can't'. Mantras can be thought or said out loud; many people believe that actually saying your mantra out loud makes it more effective, as vocalising something gives it more substance. You can also write down your chosen mantra and put it somewhere you are likely to see it, such as the kitchen or bathroom. Regularly repeating your chosen mantra will help you reaffirm your faith in yourself and your abilities.

## 41

# No need to compare

Perfectionism can be a positive thing — the desire to do better. But continually striving for a perceived version of perfection can stop you from being happy with who you already are and from seeing all the positive things you already achieve. One of the most common perfectionist tendencies is to compare yourself with others. This may take the form of direct comparison, such as 'Thomas is more successful in his job than I am' or of general comparison along the lines of 'I wish I could be more like Eve'. Either way, in seeing others as somehow better than you, you are moving your focus away from your positives. In trying to be like other people, you stop yourself from being the best version of you. Try instead to think about what areas of your life you would like to improve, and work on those areas without comparing with others, whilst recognising your strong points.

# Be assertive

When we lack confidence, it can seem like the easier option to bow to the wishes of others and say 'yes' to everything, even if you are really not happy with the situation. Though it seems like the simplest option, doing this in fact negatively affects your confidence, as you are essentially telling yourself that the wishes of others are more important than your own. Being assertive doesn't have to mean being aggressive. The main thing is that you realise your own needs are as important as everybody else's.

Try out these simple scenarios: your boss asks you to take on a new project when you are already overworked and you know that you will not be able to finish it to the necessary standard. Instead of taking it on because you think it is the correct thing to do, explain the situation to your boss, so that a solution can be found. Your friend asks you to go out, saying you will enjoy it. You know that what you really want today is to stay at home and watch a film. Instead of going out to please your friend, talk to them and let them know that you are not in the mood, and that you will see them soon for another event. The likelihood is that they will appreciate your honesty.

# Say it like you mean it

The tone of voice you adopt when speaking to people will show whether you feel confident or not. If you speak in a way which makes it obvious to the listener that you are nervous, such as in a high-pitched, broken tone, or by speaking too quickly or quietly, they will most likely not take you as seriously. Adopting a deeper, slower, more even tone of voice shows that you feel calm and self-assured, and that you know what you are talking about. This is particularly useful when speaking in public, for example when giving a presentation at work.

# CONSIDER THERAPIES

Complementary therapies are widely available and can be an excellent way to combat confidence issues, whilst giving you some 'me time' and helping you to relax.

44

# Feel better with acupressure

Acupressure is a part of traditional Chinese medicine and has been practised for many centuries. Similar to acupuncture, but without the use of needles, this gentle therapy involves applying pressure to certain pressure points to promote the free flow of energy or 'qi' through the body. Acupressure is known to help relieve muscle tension and boost circulation, both of which will leave you feeling calmer. You can go to a practitioner for acupressure or use simple acupressure techniques at home. There are many books available on the subject, or you can find tutorials online.

# Try EFT

EFT or emotional freedom techniques use tapping to unlock blocked energy, therefore improving health and well-being. Like acupuncture and acupressure, the techniques are based on the idea of 'qi' or energy moving through 'meridians' in the body, with blockages in these meridians causing illness and emotional problems. With EFT, you hold on to the negative emotion or thought which is blocking you whilst tapping on the relevant body point, then you do the same again, only this time using a positive statement to replace the negative thought. EFT can easily be tried at home, with online tutorials and illustrations readily available.

# Try the Alexander Technique

The Alexander Technique is a method developed by Frederick Matthias Alexander, an actor who realised the tension in his muscles was getting in the way of him performing at his best. He discovered that this was due to a stress reaction causing his body to adopt unnatural posture. The technique is a series of simple posture exercises which help you re-learn your natural, comfortable posture. Going to an Alexander Technique specialist will help you stand straight and tall, looking and feeling ready to take on whatever life throws at you – a definite confidence booster.

# Enjoy mood-boosting aromas

Aromatherapy uses essential oils to help calm or stimulate the mind and body. For a feel-good boost, try using stimulating oils such as geranium, rosemary or peppermint, or uplifting scents such as rose, bergamot or neroli. These can be used traditionally for massage, steam inhalation or as bath oils, but they can also be used around your home or workplace to help bring you back to yourself through the day. Try sprinkling some drops on a pomander to hang in your wardrobe, or using your favourite oil on some unscented potpourri.

## 48

# A good rub down

There is no denying that a good massage leaves you feeling more relaxed and ready to face new challenges. As well as promoting healthy blood flow and relaxing the muscles, helping you to adopt a more positive posture and giving you energy to accomplish your goals, being massaged gives you time to just focus on you. Look up a local massage therapist, or ask a friend or partner to give your shoulders, back or feet a calming, soothing rub. Alternatively, you can try self-massage on your hands, feet, legs or scalp. Using aromatherapy oils such as lavender or neroli will make this experience even more calming, and help you de-stress.

## 49

# Choose super supplements

As an extra way to bring your mood up, supplements can be very helpful. If you talk to someone at your local health food shop or natural pharmacy, they will be able to advise. The most effective herbal supplements for confidence are those which calm the mind and ease feelings of anxiety and stress. Two very popular remedies are passiflora (passion flower) and valerian. These are widely available and can be taken as a tincture or a tablet, or drunk as an infusion.

## 50

# And finally...
# seeking medical advice

If your confidence issues are having a negative effect on your day-to-day life, it is worth speaking to your doctor about it. Although complementary therapies can help a great deal, some situations need a firmer hand and sometimes low self-confidence is a sign of more serious issues. It may be that your doctor recommends a talking therapy such as CBT (cognitive behavioural therapy), or medication, to help you get to a better place. Remember, the doctor is there to help you, not to judge; tell them everything and that way they will be able to give you the best possible advice.

# Notes

.....................................................................
.....................................................................
.....................................................................
.....................................................................
.....................................................................
.....................................................................
.....................................................................
.....................................................................
.....................................................................
.....................................................................
.....................................................................
.....................................................................
.....................................................................
.....................................................................
.....................................................................

# 50 TIPS
## TO HELP YOU
# DE-STRESS

Anna Barnes

# 50 TIPS TO HELP YOU DE-STRESS

## Anna Barnes

ISBN: 978-1-84953-402-4

Hardback

£5.99

No matter how hard we try, there are times for all of us when the stresses and strains of daily life start to pile up. This book of simple, easy-to-follow tips gives you the tools and techniques you need to recognise your stress triggers and learn to take life as it comes, with a calm and balanced outlook.

# 50 TIPS
## TO HELP YOU
# SLEEP WELL

Anna Barnes

# 50 TIPS TO HELP YOU SLEEP WELL

## Anna Barnes

ISBN: 978-1-84953-401-7

Hardback

£5.99

There are times for all of us when, no matter how many sheep we have counted, falling asleep just isn't as easy as it should be. This book of simple, easy-to-follow tips provides you with the tools and techniques needed to understand your sleep patterns, and to make changes that will steer you on the path towards restful sleep.

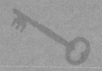

If you're interested in finding out more about our books,
find us on Facebook at **Summersdale Publishers**
and follow us on Twitter at **@Summersdale**.

# www.summersdale.com